Effortless Fat Burning: The Ultimate Cookbook for Losing Weight - Abs Are Made in the Kitchen, Not the Gym

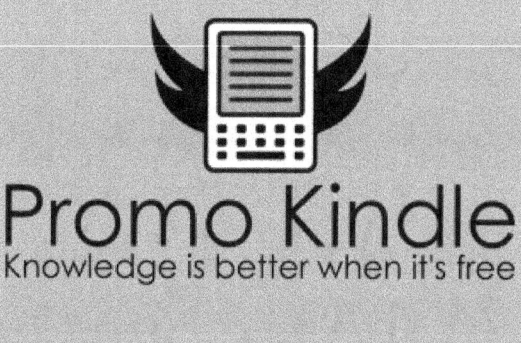

Table of Contents

BlackBerry Thyme

Ingredients:
- 1 qt. fresh blackberries
- 1 T thyme leaves
- 2 tsp sugar
- 1 T lemon juice
- 1 sourdough baguette
- 2 T butter
- 2 containers plain nonfat yogurt

Directions:

I. Stir everything but baguette and butter
II. Slice baguette and spread butter on then add the blackberry spread and serve with yogurt

Shake and hummus

Ingredients:

- 1 ½ C raspberries
- ½ C shredded kale
- 1 C ice
- ¾ C plain yogurt
- ½ banana
- 2 T honey
- 1 T almond butter
- 1 T het germ

Directions:

I. Blend well until smooth and serve
II. Serve with Hummus sandwich

Tuna White Bean Crostino

Ingredients:
- 1 can white beans
- 2 T lemon juice
- 1 T chopped parsley
- ¼ tsp salt and pepper to taste

Directions:

I.   4 slices whole wheat bread to baking sheet and divide salad over each of the slices of bread and add fontine cheese over them,

II. Broil for 2-3 minutes

Ingredients:

- 1 lbs. chicken breast
- ¼ tsp salt and pepper to taste
- 1 T olive oil
- 1 C lima beans
- ½ C corn
- 1 pint grape tomatoes
- 100 calorie whole wheat bread or roll

Directions:

I. Season and cook chicken with olive oil over skillet or grille until cooked thoroughly. Add in the lima beans and corn and serve with roll. Lemon wedges to garnish

Fried Rice

Ingredients:
- 2 T vegetable oil
- 2 C brown rice
- 2 eggs, beaten
- 2 C coleslaw mix
- 1 C shelled edamame
- 2 T soy sauce
- 1 T chile garlic sauce
- ¼ C cilantro leaves
- ¼ C chopped peanuts

Directions:

I. Heat your vegetables in a skillet with the oil and add rice cooking for about a minute
II. Stir in your eggs for about 30 seconds, and sauce.
III. Serve with cilantro and chopped peanuts

Salmon with greens

Ingredients:

- 3 T maple syrup
- 2 T vinegar
- 1 T lemon juice
- 1 T Dijon mustard
- 1 T chopped shallot
- ¼ tsp salt and pepper to taste
- 2 T olive oil
- 2 tsp. rosemary
- 4 oz. salmon fillets
- 1 C baby spinach
- ½ C shelled edamame
- ½ C red bell peppers
- ¼ C chopped almonds

Directions:

I.   Add your first five ingredients and stir in saucepan
II. For your dressing stir 2 T syrup with the olive oil and set aside
III. For your glaze heat the rest of the syrup and reduce heat for about 5 minutes uncovered and remove from heat, add in rosemary
IV. Get your broiler heated up and add the salmon and brush with glaze. Broil for about 4-5 minutes on each side

Baked Omelette

Ingredients:
- 2 T butter
- ½ C bell peppers
- ½ C chopped mushrooms
- ½ C sliced zucchini
- 1/3 C onion, chopped
- ½ tsp basil
- Salt and pepper to taste
- 3 T tomato sauce
- 10 egg whites
- 5 eggs
- ¼ C water
- ¼ C mozzarella cheese
- 2 T parmesan cheese

Directions:

I.   Preheat your oven to 400 degrees, and coat your baking dish
II.   In a skillet melt the butter and add vegetables, onions and seasonings and cook for about 5-6 minutes, and add your pepper
III. Remove skillet from the heat and stir in your tomato sauce
IV.   In a separate mixing bowl, whisk together egg whites eggs and water, add in salt
V.   Pour egg mixture into baking dish and bake for 7-10 minutes
VI.   Mix cheese in a smaller bowl, separately
VII. Cut your lengths into squares or triangles and add vegetables and cheese and fold into omelets.
VIII. Add extra tomato sauce garnish to taste

Strawberry Citrus Chicken

Ingredients:
- Chicken breasts, sliced
- 1 can chicken broth
- 2 ½ C strawberries
- 1/3 C orange juice
- 2 T salad oil
- 2 tsp shredded lemon peel
- 1 T lemon juice
- 1 tsp sugar
- ½ tsp chili powder
- Salt and pepper to taste
- 6 C spinach
- ¼ C chopped almonds

Directions:

I. Season chicken with salt and pepper, and pour broth into saucepan

II. Cook chicken in saucepan bringing it to a boil, then simmer for about 16-20 minutes, remove chicken and cool

III. Add the other remaining ingredients to food processor and blend well,

IV. Move everything into a saucepan and boil, then simmer for 5 minutes

V. Slice chicken breasts, and toss with greens and strawberries

VI. Drizzle sauce over salad with almonds

Whole Wheat Pasta with Ricotta veggies

Ingredients:

- 1 pkg. penne pasta
- 2 ½ C broccoli
- 1 ½ C asparagus, chopped
- 1 C light ricotta cheese
- 1 T dried basil
- 4 tsp dried thyme
- 1 T olive oil
- 1 T minced garlic
- Salt and pepper to taste
- 2 tomatoes, diced
- 2 T parmesan cheese

Directions:

I.   Cook pasta, bringing to a boil
II. Add your green vegetables to pasta, strain
III. In separate bowl ad cheeses and spices, stir or tossing well
IV. Add the pasta and vegetables, to ricotta
V.   Add chopped tomatoes, and toss well sprinkle with grated cheeses

Ingredients:

- ½ medium avocadoes, seeded
- 1 T lime juice
- Salt and pepper to taste
- 2 slices whole wheat bread
- 3 T cilantro
- 2 T minced garlic
- 1 can black beans, rinsed, and drained
- 1 can chipotle pepper in adobe sauce
- 2 tsp adobe sauce
- 1 tsp ground cumin
- 1 egg, beaten
- 1 tomato, chopped

Directions:

I. Mash your avocado, and stir in line juice, season with salt and pepper
II. Add bread, torn apart into food processor and crate crumbs, then chill
III. Add cilantro and garlic into food processor and process until well chopped
IV. Add everything but the egg and run processor again until well chopped
V. Bring processed mixture to eggs and blend, creating patties
VI. Grill patties over medium heat, turning or flipping once or twice
VII. Serve with tomatoes and guacamole over patties

Thai Broccoli Wraps

Ingredients:

- 12 oz. chicken breast strips
- ¼ tsp garlic salt
- 1/8 tsp pepper
- Cooking spray
- ½ tsp ginger
- 3 T creamy peanut butter
- 1 T soy sauce
- ½ tsp minced garlic
- Wheat tortillas

Directions:

I. Season your chicken with the salt and garlic and cook over medium heat for a few minutes. Add your broccoli and remaining ingredients
II. In separate saucepan add your peanut butter, water and the soy sauce along with minced garlic. Simmer until smooth saucy.
III. Add sauce to tortilla shells and spread on tortillas, add chicken and vegetables and wrap

Quinoa and Avocadoes

Ingredients:

- ½ C Quinoa
- 1 C water
- 2 tomatoes, chopped
- ½ C shredded spinach
- 1/3 C chopped onion
- 2 T lemon juice
- 2 T olive oil
- ½ tsp salt and pepper to taste
- Spinach leaves
- 2 avocadoes, pitted, sliced
- 1/3 C crumbled feta cheese

Directions:

I.   Bring Quinoa to a steady boil and the lower to a simmer, covered for about 15 minutes.
II. In separate bowl stir the quinoa, and vegetables
III. In a separate smaller bowl whisk your liquids, and add in quinoa
IV. Add spinach to your plate and serve sliced avocadoes, quinoa and feta cheese.

Fat Burning Smoothies

Apple Cider Tummy Fat burner

Ingredients:
- Apple cored
- /4 pecans
- 1 C coconut milk
- 4 ice cubes
- 1 T vanilla protein powder
- T coconut butter
- 1 tsp cinnamon
- 1 tsp nutmeg
- Stevia

Directions:

I.   Blend and serve

Berry Smoothie

Ingredients:
- 2 C strawberries
- 1 C blueberries
- 1 C cherries
- 1 C milk
- 1 oz whey protein

Directions:

I.   Blend and serve

Green Tea Berry Smoothie

Ingredients:

- Green Tea
- 2 C blueberries
- 12 oz. fat free yogurt
- ½ C ice cube
- 2 T almonds
- 2 T ground flax seeds

Directions:

I.   Blend and serve

Vanilla Coconut Smoothie

Ingredients:
- 8 oz. coconut milk
- 2 eggs
- 1 T EVOO
- Frozen banana
- ¼ C berries
- 1 T whey protein powder

Directions:

I.   Blend and serve

Chocolate covered berry Smoothie

Ingredients:
- 1 scoop whey protein powder
- Chitosan
- ½ C ice
- ½ banana
- 1 C water
- ½ C frozen blueberries
- 1 tsp unsweetened cocoa
- ½ pack of milled flaxseed

Directions:

I.   Blend and serve

Pomegranate Smoothie

Ingredients:
- 1 12 C frozen berries
- 1 C pomegranate juice
- 1 pomegranate
- 1 oz. whey protein powder
- 1 T honey
- 1 banana

Directions:

I.   Blend and serve

Sleep weight Loss smoothie

Ingredients:

- 1 C cherry juice
- ½ C soy milk
- ½ banana
- ¼ tsp pure vanilla extract
- Ice

Directions:

I.   Blend and serve

Tropical Tummy tucking Smoothie

Ingredients:
- 6 oz. fat free Greek Yogurt
- ¾ C coconut milk
- 1 banana
- 1 C spinach
- ¾ C fresh pineapple chunks
- Ice
- 2 T shredded coconut

Directions:

I.   Blend or process until smooth

Mango Smoothie

Ingredients:
- 1 C chopped mango
- Ice
- ½ C low fat milk
- ¼ C Fat free yogurt
- 1 T honey

Directions:

I.   Blend and serve

Protein Smoothie

Ingredients:
- 1 apple
- 12 oz. almond milk
- 1 oz. vanilla protein powder
- 1 tsp cinnamon
- 1 tsp nutmeg
- Ice

Directions:

I.   Blend and serve

Just Peachy Smoothie

Ingredients:
- 2 ½ C peaches
- 2 C soy milk
- 3 T almond butter
- 1 tsp cinnamon
- Ice
- Slivered almonds

Directions:

I.   Blend and serve

Greek Yogurt Smoothie

Ingredients:
- 1 banana
- ¾ C frozen strawberries
- ½ C almond milk
- ½ C Greek yogurt

Directions:

I.   Blend and serve

Cucumber Fresh Smoothie

Ingredients:
- 2 cucumbers, diced
- 1 Greek Yogurt container
- 2 tsp agave nectar
- Mint leaves
- ½ lime, juice
- Ice
- Black pepper to taste

Directions:

I. Blend and serve

www.ingramcontent.com/pod-product-compliance
Lightning Source LLC
Chambersburg PA
CBHW070527290526
45790CB00003B/1331